Radia BENYAHIA
Chahira MAZOUZI

Breast microcalcifications: from diagnosis to sampling

Radia BENYAHIA
Chahira MAZOUZI

Breast microcalcifications: from diagnosis to sampling

Investigation of breast microcalcifications

ScienciaScripts

Imprint
Any brand names and product names mentioned in this book are subject to trademark, brand or patent protection and are trademarks or registered trademarks of their respective holders. The use of brand names, product names, common names, trade names, product descriptions etc. even without a particular marking in this work is in no way to be construed to mean that such names may be regarded as unrestricted in respect of trademark and brand protection legislation and could thus be used by anyone.

Cover image: www.ingimage.com

This book is a translation from the original published under ISBN 978-620-6-70054-8.

Publisher:
Sciencia Scripts
is a trademark of
Dodo Books Indian Ocean Ltd. and OmniScriptum S.R.L publishing group

120 High Road, East Finchley, London, N2 9ED, United Kingdom
Str. Armeneasca 28/1, office 1, Chisinau MD-2012, Republic of Moldova, Europe
Printed at: see last page
ISBN: 978-620-7-03553-3

BREAST
MICROCALCIFICATIONS

PREFACE

Microcalcifications are calcium deposits in breast tissue detected by mammography. Although most microcalcifications are not associated with breast cancer, their presence can reveal an incipient lesion. Their early detection is essential for effective diagnosis and treatment of breast cancer.

This book has been designed to provide you with a practical resource on breast microcalcifications, from their detection to their removal. You will find detailed information on the different imaging modalities used to detect microcalcifications, as well as the radiological characteristics of benign and malignant lesions.

We have also included a second chapter on percutaneous sampling of microcalcifications. We hope that this book will help you to better understand breast microcalcifications and to improve your skills in breast radiology.

Co-author: Mazouzi Chahira

1. Introduction

Mammary microcalcifications are calcium-toned images with a diameter of less than 1mm found on mammography. They may be related to benign or malignant lesions.
In 70% of cases, microcalcifications indicate a benign pathology.
The discovery of micro-calcifications requires a precise study of their radiological aspects in order to approach their benign or malignant nature, avoiding over-diagnosis and therefore over-treatment for benign lesions and appropriate and optimal management for malignant lesions.

2. Physicochemical aspects

There are two physicochemical types of microcalcifications (1) :

Type I: corresponds to calcium oxalate weddelite crystals, always associated with benign pathology (figure 1 a); these benign calcifications, of particular shape (octahedrons), result from the precipitation of intra-cystic calcium. Their pyramidal shape makes them birefringent and their histological detection is based on examination of the slides under polarised light. In mammography, their particular square or diamond-shaped morphology can be detected if the microcalcifications are dense and large (Figure 1).

Type II: this is the most frequent type, corresponding to calcium phosphate, non-crystalline, when encountered in benign and malignant pathology.

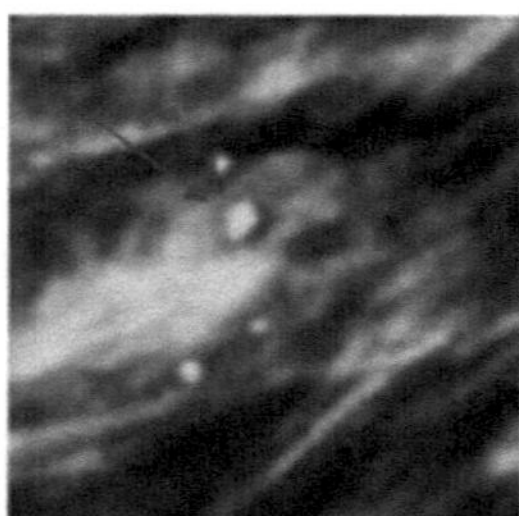

Figure 1: weddelite crystal-type breast microcalcifications

3. Pathophysiology

The shape and distribution of microcalcifications are linked :

➤ The physiopathological process that gave rise to them, i.e. cell necrosis and secretory phenomena (stasis and calcium precipitation);

➤ And where they were formed.

Mammary micro-calcifications develop in various components of the mammary gland:

➤ Connective tissue: Related to the fibrosis and inflammation of benign or scarring mastopathies and the reactive stroma of cancer;

➤ The epithelial lining of the galactophoric duct: For benign proliferative mastopathies of the epithelium (HCA with or without atypia) and also in malignant proliferative mastopathies (ductal carcinoma in situ or infiltrating);

➢ Galactophore ducts: by stagnation of secretions leading to calcium precipitation in fibrocystic dysplasia or by tumour compression of the duct (ductal carcinoma in situ or infiltrating).

4. Anatomical reminder

The mammary gland is a paired gland of ectodermal embryological origin, located on the anterior surface of the thorax, whose development is influenced by hormones and age.

The mammary gland is made up of connective support tissue, breast tissue and adipose tissue. The glandular tissue is made up of 15 to 20 lobes, each lobe contains lobules and each lobule is made up of acini, which communicate with each other via the mammary duct (Figure 2).

The ductus galactophoricus terminates at the areola and then undergoes a dichotomous division to give the ductulo-lobular terminal unit, which is the functional unit of the mammary gland (2).

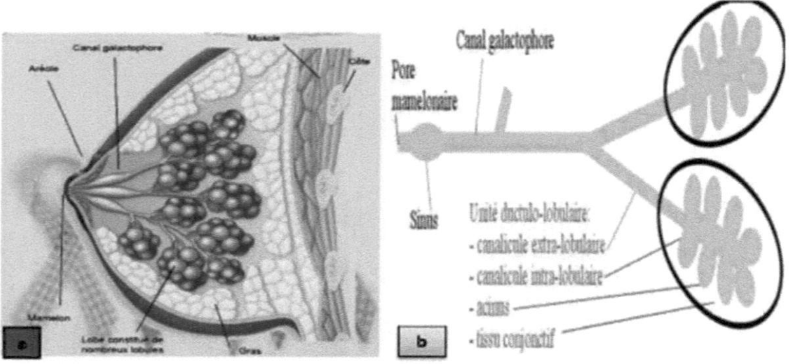

Figure 2.

a. Schematic sagittal section of the mammary gland b. Schematic image of the ductulo-lobular terminal unit

5. Circumstances of discovery

The clinical circumstances in which microcalcifications are discovered are either (Figure 3):

- ➢ Following a screening mammogram ;

- ➢ Or at the time of a diagnostic mammogram, carried out to explore a clinical abnormality of the breast such as :

- Retraction of the nipple;
- The appearance of a mass ;
- There may even be a discharge from the nipple.

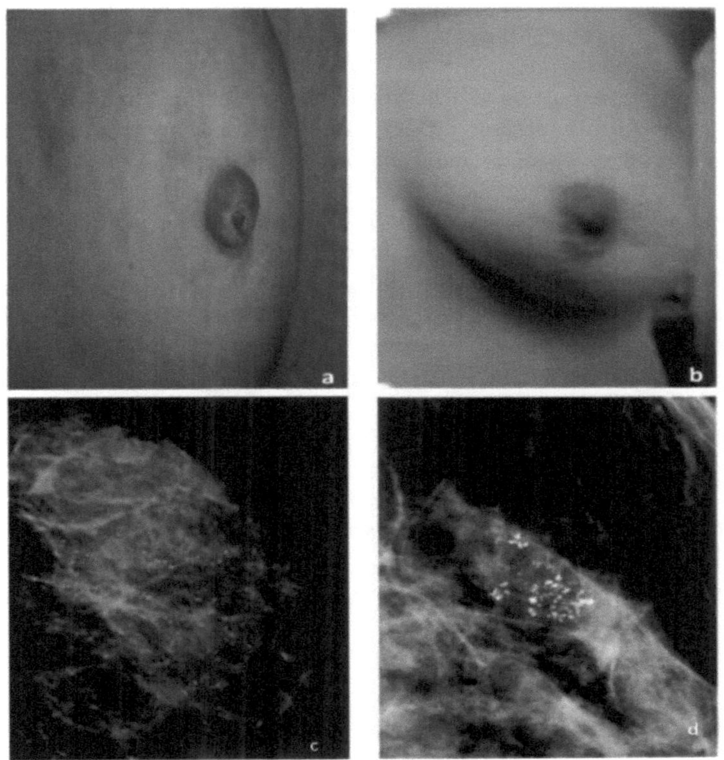

Figure 3
a. Nipple eczema
b. Normal breast
c. Suspected extensive microcalcifications
d. Coarse microcalcifications grouped in suspicious foci

6. Exploration techniques

6.1. Mammography

Mammography is the reference examination in breast imaging, enabling the detection of breast lesions (masses, calcifications, architectural distortions). The detection of micro-calcifications and their characterisation must be as accurate as possible in order to optimise their management; this requires quality control of the mammographic chain (mammography, reprogramming and negatoscope, etc.).

The mammography technique must be rigorous, meeting multiple technical requirements such as contrast and radiation dose.
Finally, the positioning of the patient and the basic incidences and additional images must be perfectly mastered in order to avoid diagnostic errors and reduce the number of images, and therefore the radiation exposure of patients.

6.1.1. Positioning

Positioning the breast is an essential stage in mammography, and the technique must be rigorous. Good positioning is the basis of a quality image. The breast must be well spread out. In order to radiograph the entire mammary gland, including the deep layers, it must meet certain criteria.

6.1.2. Basic impact

A. Front view or cranio-caudal view

Quality criteria

According to the ACR recommendations, the quality criteria for a mammographic image of the face are (Figure 5) (3, 4):

➢ A nipple at its zenith projecting outside the mammary gland, well centred in the middle of the image;
➢ Good spreading of the retroareolar fibroglandular meshwork;
➢ Visibility of retroglandular fat ;
➢ A visible pectoral in 30% to 40% of cases;
➢ Absence of skin folds.

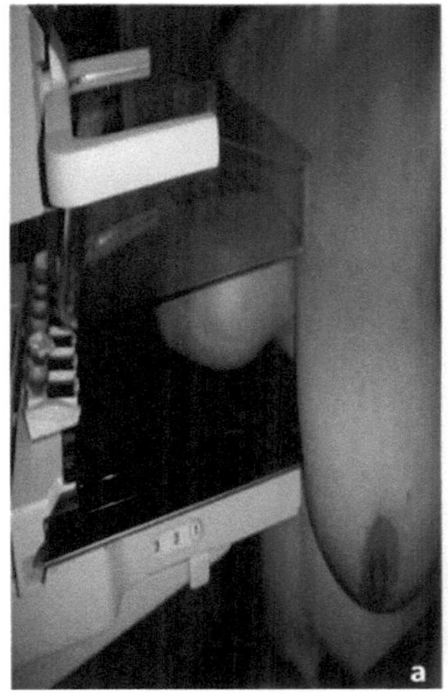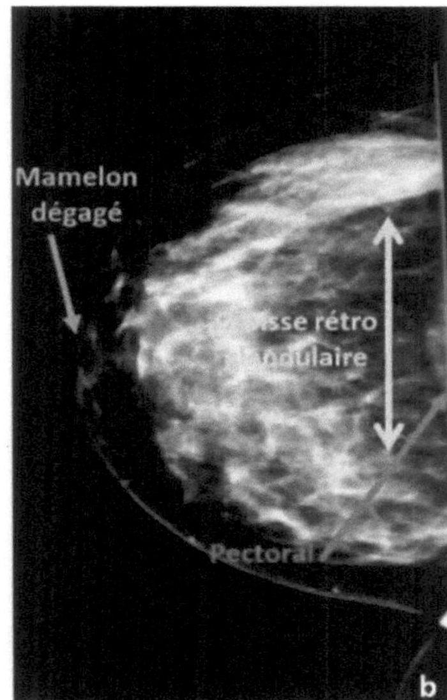

Figure 4: Frontal incidence and success criteria

B. External oblique incidence

Quality criteria

According to the ACR recommendations, these are (Figure 5):

➤ The tip of the pectoral is well spread out and visible right up to the nipple;

➤ A convex edge of the pectoral ;

➤ A nipple at its zenith projecting outside the mammary gland;

➤ Good spreading of the retroareolar fibroglandular meshwork;

➤ The visible submammary fold ;

➤ Absence of skin folds.

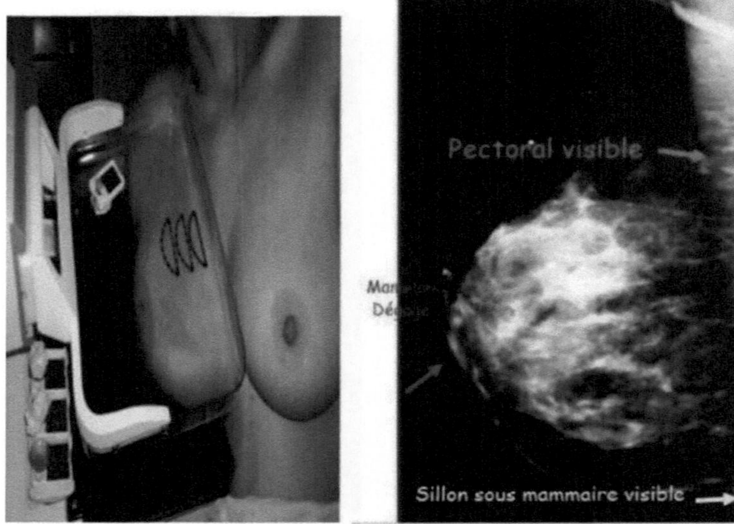

Figure 5: External oblique incidence and success criteria

6.1.3 Additional impacts (5,6)

A. Profile incidence

A.1 Quality criteria

According to the ACR recommendations, these are (Figure 6):
➤ Good spreading of the retroareolar fibroglandular meshwork;
➤ Visibility of retroglandular fat ;
➤ A thin but visible pectoral in the upper part of the image;
➤ The nipple projects outside the mammary gland;
➤ A visible submammary fold;
➤ Absence of skin folds.

A.2 Indications

➤ Better locate an anomaly detected on one of the basic incidences ;
➤ Locate an abnormality for preoperative mapping or macro biopsy under stereotaxy (7);
➤ Characterise a focus of microcalcifications (detect a horizontal sediment, typically benign "milk of calcium").

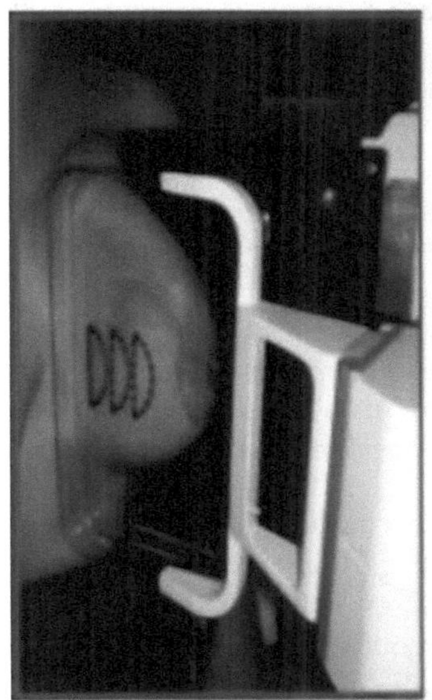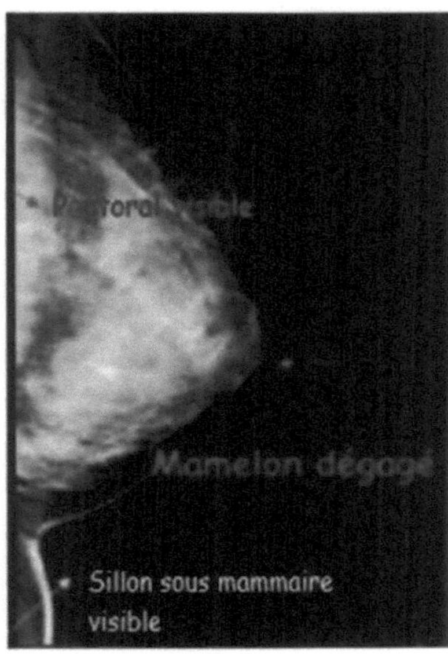

Figure 6: Profile incidence and success criteria

B. Enlarged incidence (8, 9)

The magnification effect (geometric, not digital) allows a detailed analysis of the calcification focus, i.e. its distribution and shape (figure 7).

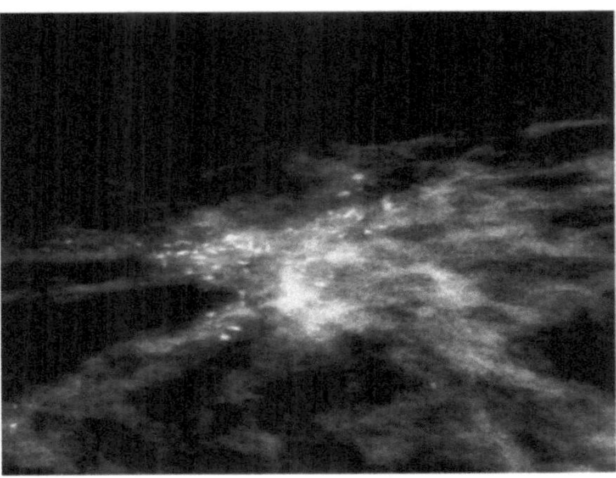

Figure 7. Magnification: Mass associated with microcalcifications

6.1.4 Indications for mammography (10, 11)

Diagnostic mammography is performed :

- To diagnose a palpable anomaly or symptom (mastodynia, inflammation, nipple discharge, skin changes, etc.);
- To make an aetiological diagnosis of a sub-clinical anomaly revealed by organised screening ;
- As part of individual screening (family history giving rise to suspicion of a genetic predisposition).

It must be preceded by an interview and a clinical examination.
It involves two or three views per breast and, in addition, any views that may prove useful for diagnosis (enlarged localized views in particular).

The aim of diagnostic mammography is to make the final diagnosis in a single session and to determine the course of action to be taken thanks to an immediate reading of the images (whether or not further investigations, samples or surgery are required).

6.1.5 Performance of mammography in detecting breast cancer

A. Sensitivity

The sensitivity of mammography is very high for radiolucent breasts, approaching 98% for fat-dense breasts (12, 13) (Figure 8).

As far as the detection of microcalcifications is concerned, even in a dense breast, the sensitivity of mammography remains high, because almost half of all cancers contain microcalcifications, and this is the tell-tale sign in 90% of insitu cancers.

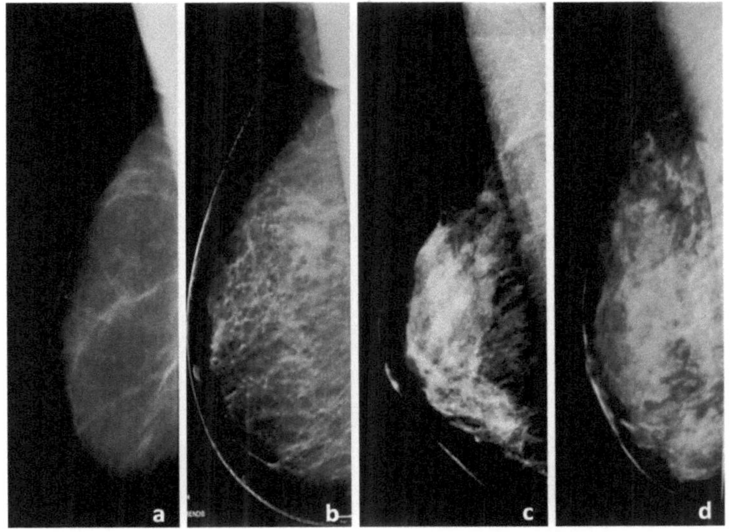

Figure 8. Breast density according to the ACR Bi-Rads® classification

a. Type a, b. Type b, c. Type c, d. Type d.

B. Specificity

The mammographic aspect is specific in a number of cases:

➤ Totally radiolucent breast with no abnormalities;
➤ Typical intra mammary node ;
➤ Typical calcified fibroadenoma ;
➤ Lipoma ;
➤ Typical hamartoma ;
➤ Typical malignant stellar image with a dense centre.

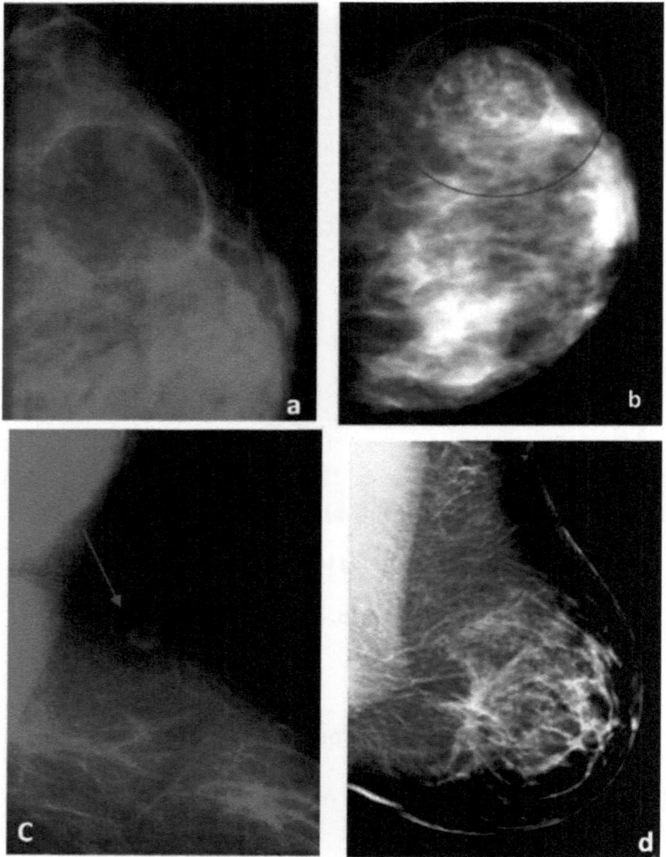

Figure 9. Specific aspects of mammographic masses
a. Lipoma, b. Hamar tome, c. Intra mammary lymph node, d. Stellate mass.

6.2   Other imaging methods

6.2.1 Breast ultrasound

Breast ultrasound has no place in the investigation of isolated microcalcifications and cannot make up for the false negatives of mammography, but it can characterise non-mass lesions and look for breast lesions that have gone undetected on mammography (14).

The ultrasound non-mass is a poorly systematised, hypoechoic, heterogeneous area with echogenic spots within it related to extensive microcalcifications on mammography (Figure 10).

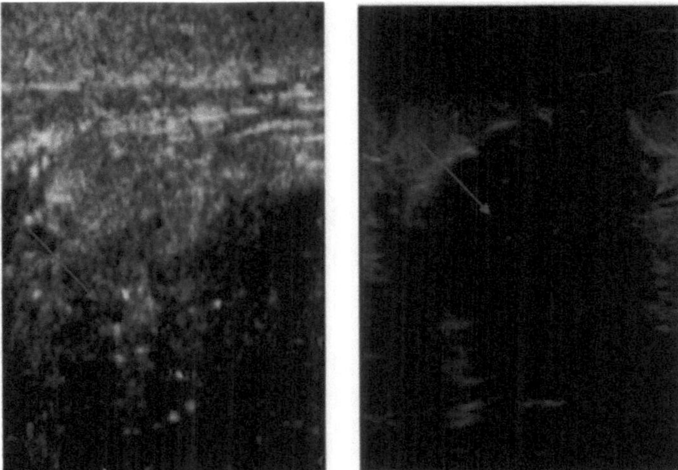

Figure 10. Ultrasound non-mass: poorly defined heterogeneous hypoechoic areas containing echogenic spots associated with microcalcifications.

6.2.2 Breast MRI

When breast microcalcifications are <u>isolated, with</u> no associated mass, overdensity or architectural distortion, breast MRI provides no additional information and is therefore negative (no morphological or haemodynamic translation of the microcalcifications) (Figure 11).

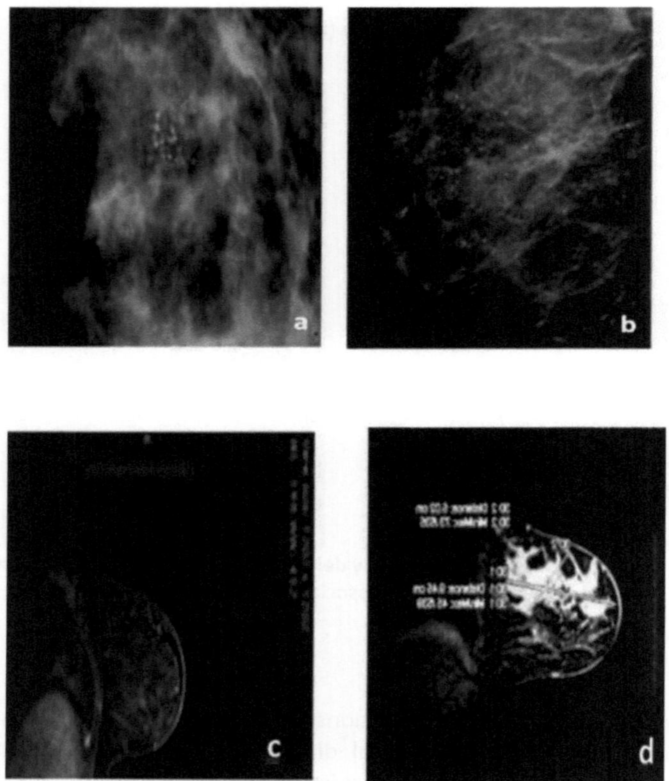

Figure 11

a. Isolated focus of microcalcification, b. Extensive microcalcifications associated with asymmetric density, c. No translation of the focus of microcalcification on MRI, d. MRI shows extensive segmental non-mass enhancement related to the microcalcifications and *overdensity.*

7   The ACR BI-RADS classification for calcifications

According to the BI-RADS classification, breast calcifications are essentially classified into three types according to their form:

➢ Typically benign calcifications;

➢ Calcifications of intermediate concern ;

➢ Calcifications with a higher probability of malignancy.

Two other criteria have been added to the description of microcalcifications: the distribution and the evolution of calcifications over time.

The final classification will be based on the most pejorative criterion, which will be used to define the course of action.

All mammographic, ultrasound and MRI abnormalities will be classified into 7 categories according to the BI-RADS system (Breast imaging reporting and data system) of the ACR (American College of Radiology)

➢ **ACR 0:** Unclassifiable image requiring further imaging

➢ **ACR 1:** No pathological calcification to describe

➢ **ACR 2 :**

❖ Annular or arciform microcalcifications, sedimented like milk of calcium, dystrophic in profile;

❖ Diffuse regular punctiform microcalcifications ;

❖ Skin and vascular calcifications ;

❖ Large rod-shaped calcifications with clear centres, parietal, calcified sutures.

➢ **ACR 3:** Regular round or punctiform microcalcifications, or very fine, few in number, in small isolated round clusters

➢ **ACR 4 :**

❖ Numerous regular punctiform microcalcifications, or grouped in clusters with irregular outlines;

❖ Numerous groupings of very fine micro-calcifications.

➢ **ACR 5 :**

❖ Vermicular, arborescent microcalcifications;

❖ Polymorphous or granular microcalcifications ;

❖ Clusters of microcalcifications of canal distribution ;

❖ Microcalcifications associated with a mass ;

❖ Grouped microcalcifications which have increased in number.

➢ **ACR 6:** Histologically proven malignancy.

8 Morphological aspects of microcalcifications and their distribution

8.1 Calcification morphologies

8.1.1 Skin calcifications

Best analysed by tangential incision, they are generally located in the under mammary fold and in the axilla, presenting as calcifications with clear centres.

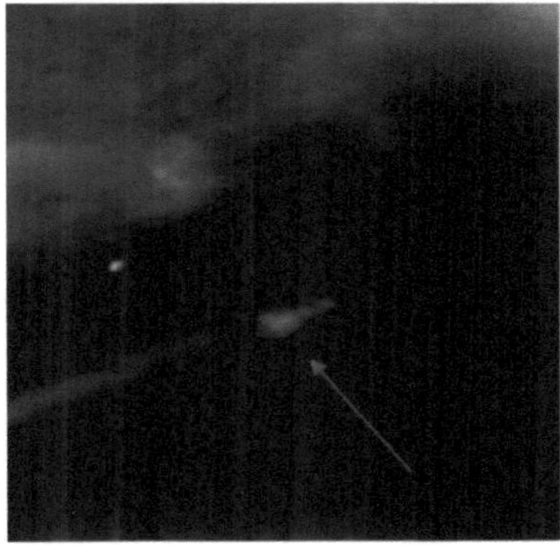

8.1.2 Vascular calcifications

Parietal vascular calcifications of atheromatous origin, linear and parallel, giving the appearance of a rail.

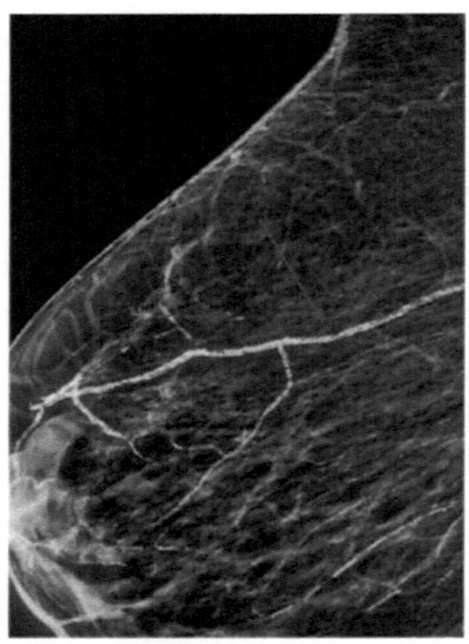

8.1.3 Coarse or coralliform calcifications

These are large calcifications measuring 2-3 mm.

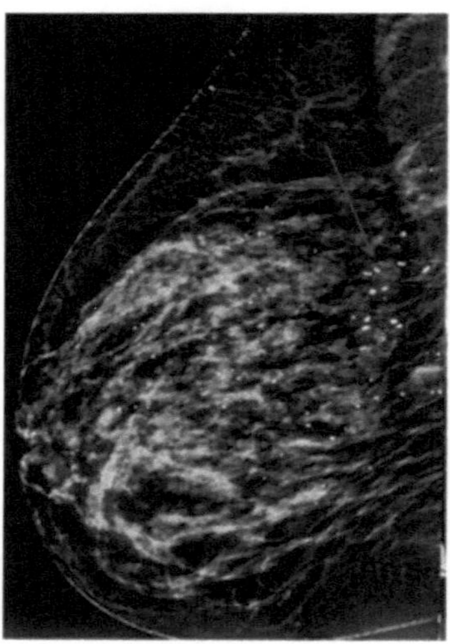

8.1.4 Large rod-shaped calcifications: distributed towards the nipple
Supra-millimetre in size, discontinuous with smooth edges, most often located in the retroareolar region secondary to chronic

galactophoritis.

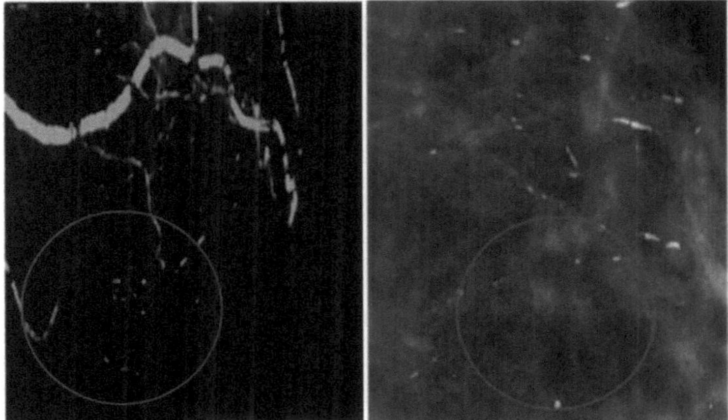

8.1.5 Eggshell calcifications

These are peripheral calcifications which surround the wall of a cyst and are also found in foci of cytosteonecrosis.

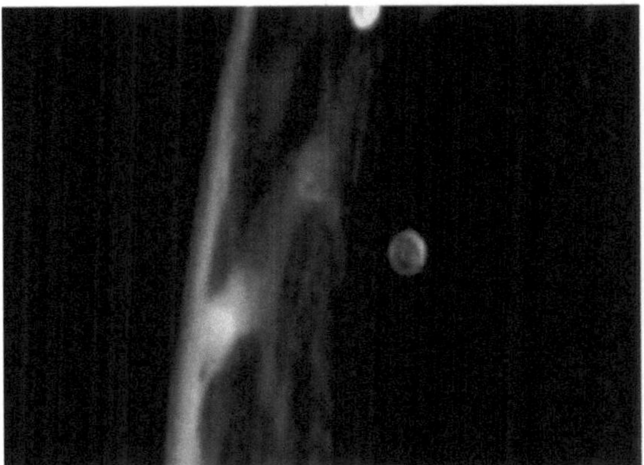

8.1.6 Round calcifications

They develop within the acini and are less than 1mm in size. They are benign if they are scattered.

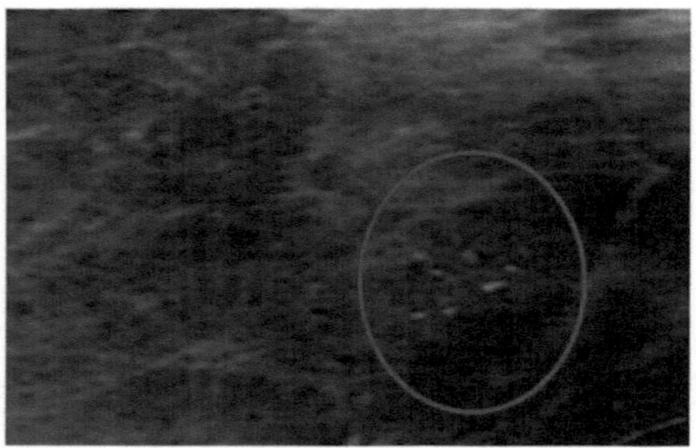

8.1.7 Calcifications with a clear centre

➤ Round or oval with a smooth surface and a light centre;
➤ Thicker-walled than eggshell calcifications;
➤ Calcification of cytosteato necrosis or calcified ductal debris.

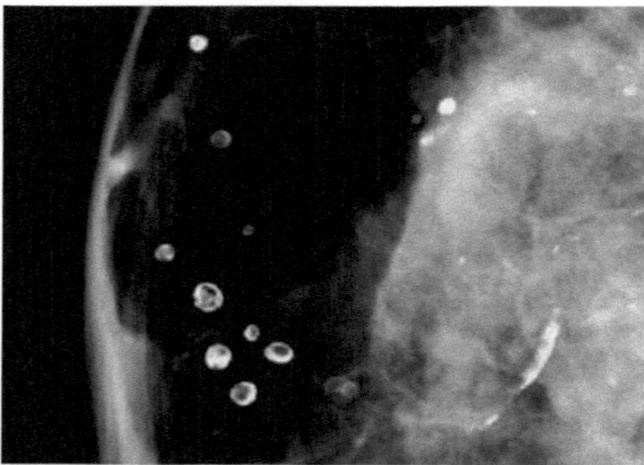

8.1.8 Calcium milk-type calcifications

They are due to calcified intra-cystic sedimentation and can be seen on the frontal view, but on the lateral view they give a semi-moon-like appearance known as a "cup of tea".

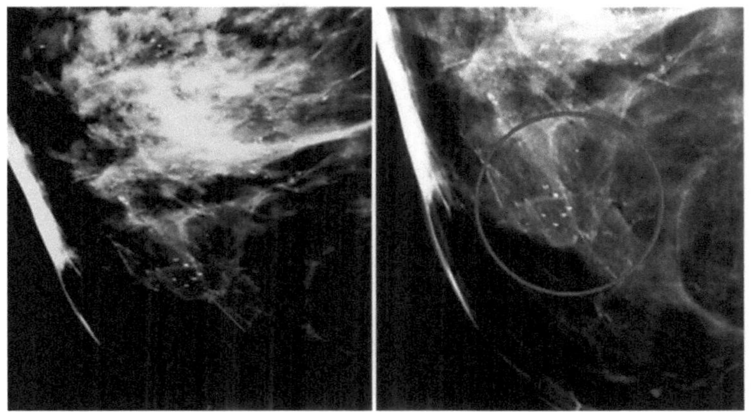

8.1.9 Amorphous, indistinct or dusty calcifications

These are calcifications that are too thin and difficult to see around.

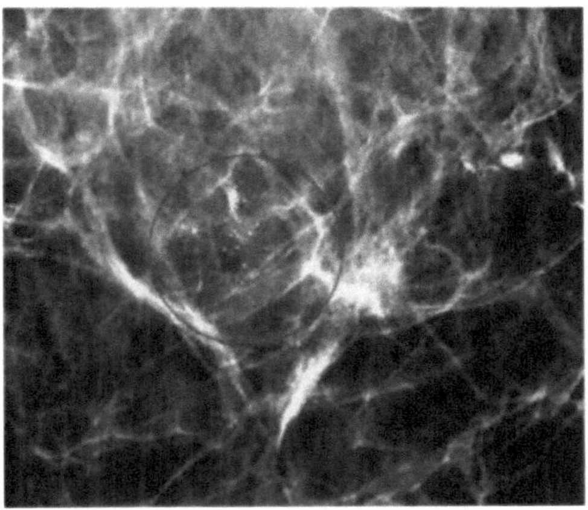

8.1.10 Coarse, heterogeneous calcifications

These calcifications vary in size and shape.

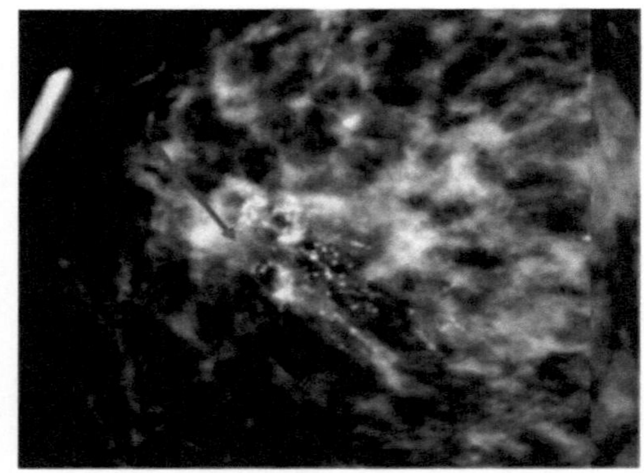

8.1.11 Fine polymorphic calcifications

These are microcalcifications with distinct, well-defined contours.

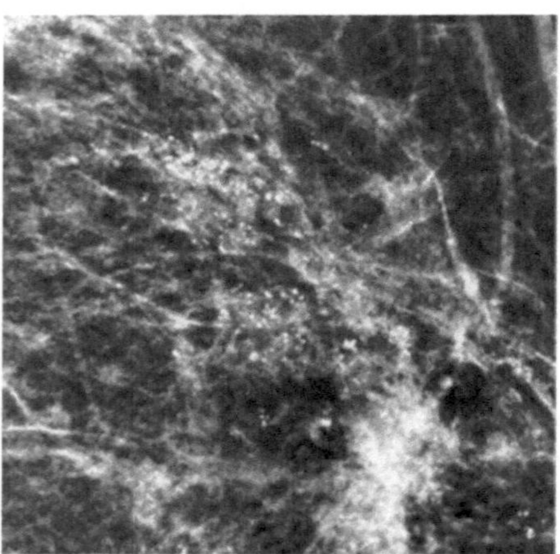

8.2 Distribution of calcifications

> Scattered, diffuse, of **interest throughout the breast**

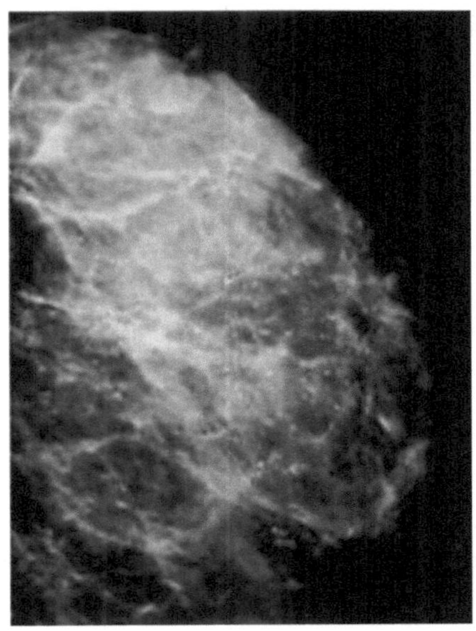

> **Regional:** occupying the whole of one quadrant or more.

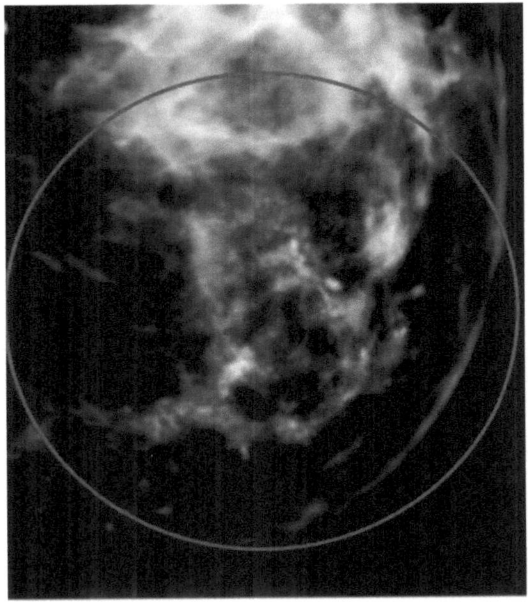

> **Grouped in clusters or foci:** These are microcalcifications of which

there are more than 5, occupying a volume of less than 1 cc.

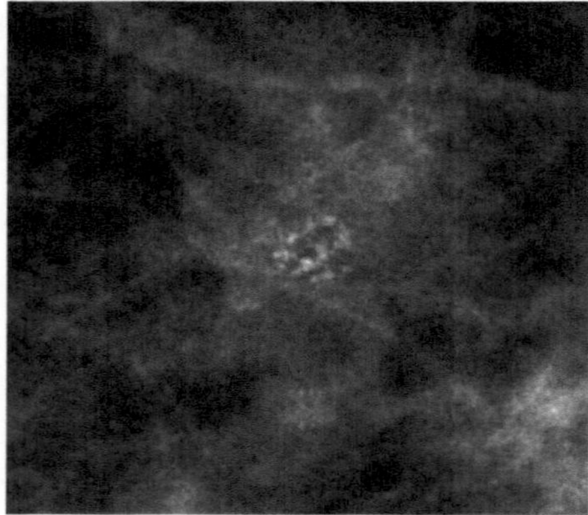

> **Linear: These are** intra-galactophoreal **calcifications.**

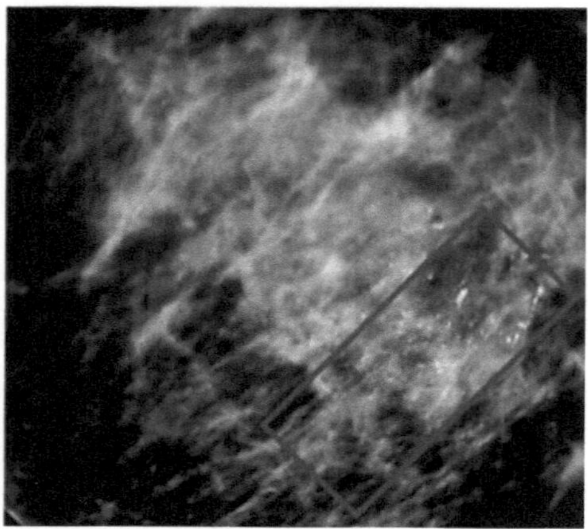

> **Segmental: these are calcifications with a triangular distribution** with a peripheral base and vertices pointing towards the nipple.

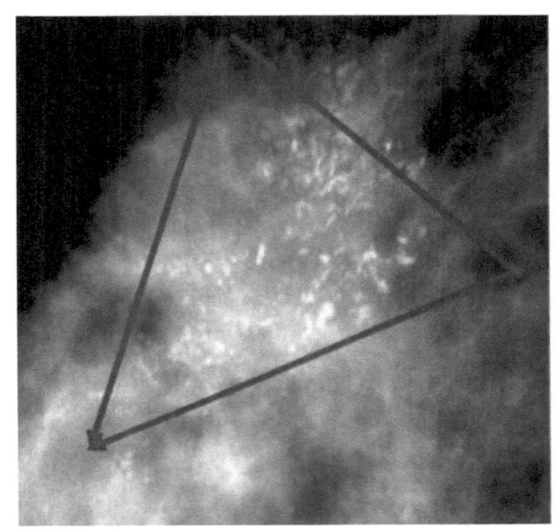

9   Conclusion

The aim of screening is to discover cancers at the sub-clinical, microcalcification stage, which is the best guarantee of conservative treatment and an excellent prognosis.

Strict quality control, perfect technique and vigilant analysis of mammographic images are the key factors in the discovery of a focus of microcalcifications.

Malignant radiological features require histological proof by macro biopsy under stereotaxis.

REFERENCES

1. Ko pa N S DB. Anatomy. histology, physiology and pathology. In: Breast imaging. 2nJed. Philadelphia. Lippincott-Raven. 1998: 3-27.
2. Heidsieck R, Laurencin G, Ponchin A, Gabbay E, Klausz R. Dual target X-ray tubes for mammographic examinations: dose reduction with image quality equivalent to that with standard mammographic tubes. [abstract]. Radiology 1991; 181 (P): 311
3. Hessler C, Bochud F, Grecescu M, Valley JF, Vauthey JL, Verdun FR. Intercomparison of screen-film pairs in mammography. J le Sein 1993; 3: 195-197
4. Hessler C, Bochud F, Valley JF, Verdun FR. Quality control in mammography. Société française de radiologie et d'imagerie médicale: Journées francophones de radiologie, cours de perfectionnement postuniversitaire. Paris, 23-27 October 1995.
5. Gwdrich WA Jr. The Cleopatra view in xeromammography: a semi-reclining position of the tail of the breast. Radiology. 1978. 128 : 811-812.
6. Emel A. Kagan C, Enrico C. Timur S. An effective way to solve cquivocal mammography findings: the rolled views. Breast Care. 2010, 5 : 241-245.
7. Pf. arson KL, Sickles EA, Frankel SD, Leung JWT. Efficacy of step-oblique mammography for confirmation and localization of densities seen on only one standard mammographie view. AJR Am J Roentgenol, 2000. 174 : 745-752.
8. Specifications for organised breast cancer screening. Journal officiel no. 295 of 21 December 2006: 278-313 (www. joumalofficiegouv. fr).
9. 276/Muntz EP. Logan WW. Focal spot size and scatter suppression in magnification mammography. AJR Am J Roentgenol, 1979. 133 : 453-459.
10. Wallyn-Moraux M. Chaveron C. Bachelle F et al. Comparative study in the analysis of microcalcification foci between geometric enlargements and digital zoom. J Radiol, 2010, 91 : 879-883
11. ChopierJ. JalaguierA. Thomassin-Naggaral. Variations of the normal breast: mammographic and echographic aspects. Encycl Med Chir (Paris). 34-800-A15.
12. American college of radiology. ACR. BI-RADS-mammography. Paris. Societe francaise de Radiologie. 2004 : 175-176.
13. Stavros AT, Thickman D. Rapp CL et al. Solid breast nodules: use of sonography to distinguish benign and malignant nodules. Radiology, 1995, 796 : 123-134
14. Rahbar G. Sie AC. Hansen GC et al. Benign versus malignant solid breast masses: US differentiation. Radiology. 1999. 213 : 889-894.

MACROBIOPSY UNDER STEREOTAXIS

PREFACE

Interventional breast imaging is an integral part of patient care and plays a significant and growing role in radiologists' work.

The advent of interventional breast imaging has made it easier to learn and master breast pathology.

Macro biopsy under stereotaxis is a technique for percutaneous sampling of breast tissue that offers a safe alternative to surgical biopsy, enabling early, rapid and accurate histological diagnosis of microcalcification sites.

This chapter is designed to present this procedure with all the steps necessary to achieve a reliable diagnosis and improve the management of breast microcalcifications.

1. Introduction

Individual screening and the introduction of mass screening for breast cancer have led to an increase in the detection of sub-clinical lesions.
Subclinical lesions in breast imaging correspond to microcalcifications, masses or architectural disorganisation.

When a mammogram reveals an abnormality, further investigations are required to confirm or rule out the malignant nature of the lesion.

Percutaneous breast sampling is often the only way to diagnose and manage breast pathology. They are a genuine alternative to surgical biopsy. Surgical biopsy for diagnostic purposes is, however, reserved for complex situations.

Percutaneous sampling, when carried out under imaging control, may be guided by ultrasound, mammography or MRI; the target is either a mass, a patch, microcalcifications or architectural distortion. Depending on the needle gauge, the procedure is referred to as microbiopsy (gauge greater than 12 gauges) or macrobiopsy (gauge less than or equal to 12 gauges) [1, 2].

2. Different methods of guiding percutaneous sampling

Interventional breast surgery is guided primarily by imaging and, if the lesion is palpable, by the clinic. For sub-clinical lesions, radiological control allows more precise targeting. The choice of radiological guidance depends on a number of factors, such as the speed of the procedure, irradiation, and better visualisation of the target. Two main guidance methods are used: mammography and ultrasound.

3. Stereotactic macrobiopsy

Stereotactic macrobiopsy by aspiration consists of removing breast tissue from an abnormality that cannot be detected by mammography. Most often, the target is a focus of microcalcifications grouped in clusters or spread out in patches in 90% of cases, but in 10% of cases the target may present as a mass, architectural distortion or asymmetry of density, which are not reflected on ultrasound [5, 10].
In macrobiopsy under stereotaxy, large-calibre needles ranging from 7 to 11 G are used. The number of specimens depends on the size of the target, its extent and the calibre of needle used (Figures 1).

Thus, for a sub-centimetre image (mass or focus), the biopsy is representative if it removes at least 50% of the target.
The ideal number of samplings with a needle greater than or equal to 10G would be 12 [10].

Macrobiopsy is a procedure that must be discussed and approved at a multidisciplinary consultation meeting (RCP).

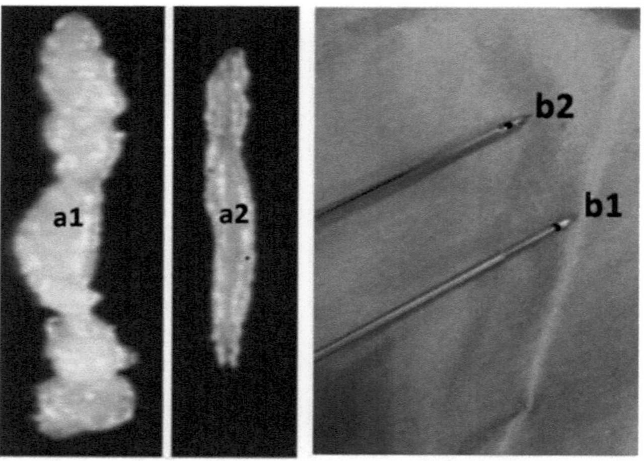

Figure 1. a: 7 Gauge (al), 10 Gauge (a2) tissue samples b : 7 Gauge (bl), 10G (b2)

needles

4. The stereotactic biopsy procedure

4.1. Principle of the technique

The principle of stereotaxy, whether using an add-on system or a dedicated digitised table, is to determine the spatial co-ordinates of an infra-clinical target from two identical but opposite angles; in other words, to specify the position of a target on two mammographic images taken with an angulation generally of the order of +15° and -15°, making it possible to calculate its location in space. Once the location of the target in the breast has been calculated, the biopsy needle is inserted into the correct position using a mechanical system [12, 13, 14].

In stereotaxy, two types of device are available, which have the same principle of use but differ in the way they operate (Figure 2).

- ➢ One uses a dedicated digitised table where the patient is placed in procubitus position;
- ➢ The other is an add-on system that can be fitted to a digital mammography unit for 2D or 3D macrobiopsy, with the patient in a sitting or lateral decubitus position.

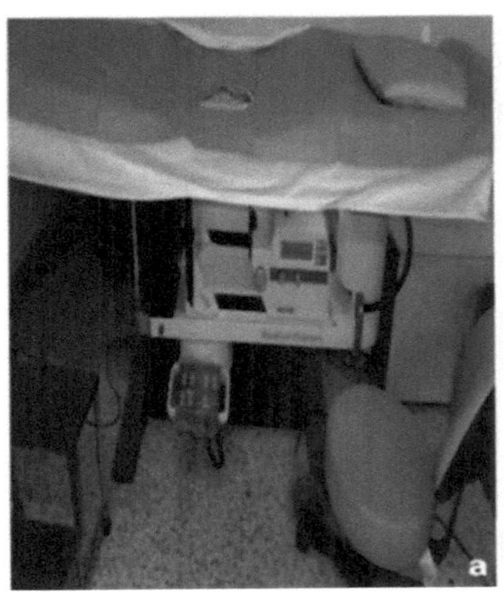
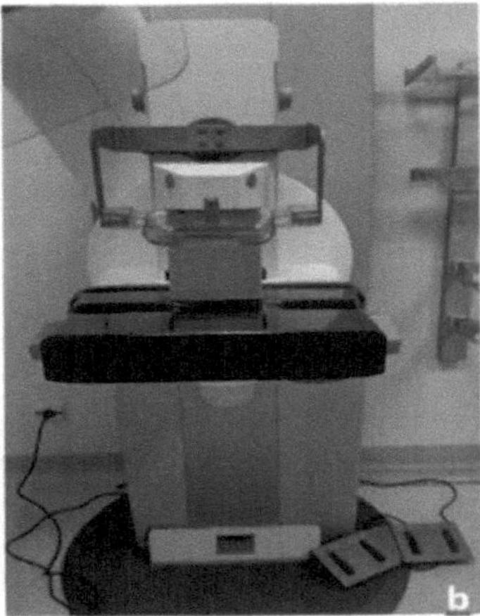

Figure 2: Dedicated digitised table for stereotactic macrobiopsy (a); 3D mammography (tomography) with add-on stand for stereotactic macrobiopsy (b).

4.2. Stereotaxis procedure

The stereotactic macrobiopsy of the breast is performed as an outpatient procedure under local anaesthetic.

The patient is placed either in the procubitus position, or in the sitting position, or lateral position for the biopsy, which is performed on an add-on stand.

The vertical or lateral approach is then chosen, taking into account the shortest route to the target. When using a dedicated digitised table

The examination in both systems begins with :

Compression of the breast and centring of the target in the middle of the paddle opening (Figure 3).

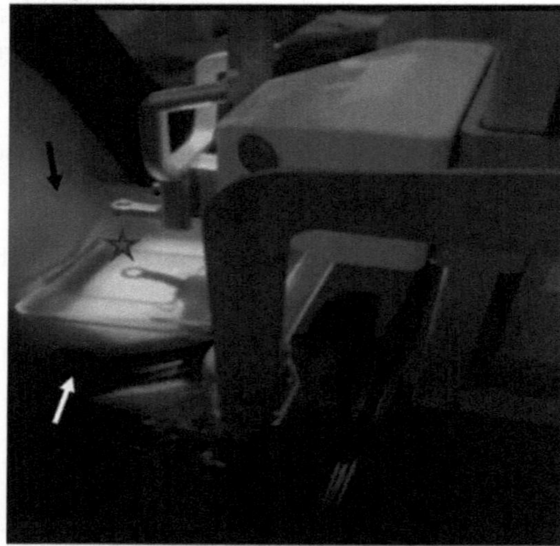

Figure 3: Centring the target: breast (black arrow) compressed by the compression paddle (white arrow); centring hole for the needle (star).

> A first click at a 0° angle (scout view) is taken, showing the lesion to be sampled in the field of view (opening of the pallet (figure 4 a);

> Once the lesion has been centred, two stereotactic images are taken (generally at +15 and -15°) (Figure 4 b).

> Position the markers in the centre of the lesion to be biopsied;

> Disinfection of the skin inside the biopsy window ;

> Local anaesthesia in the centre of the lesion;

> Positioning the needle on its support ;

> Skin incision at reference point ;

> The needle is inserted through the skin incision.

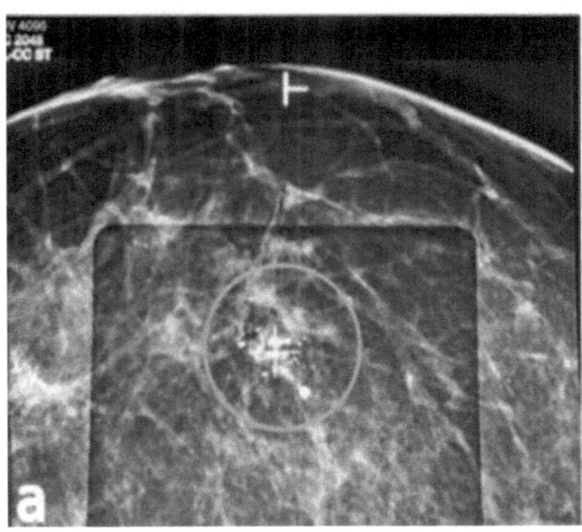

Figure 4 a. Stereotactic "scout view" views of a focus of microcalcifications in the 0° position.

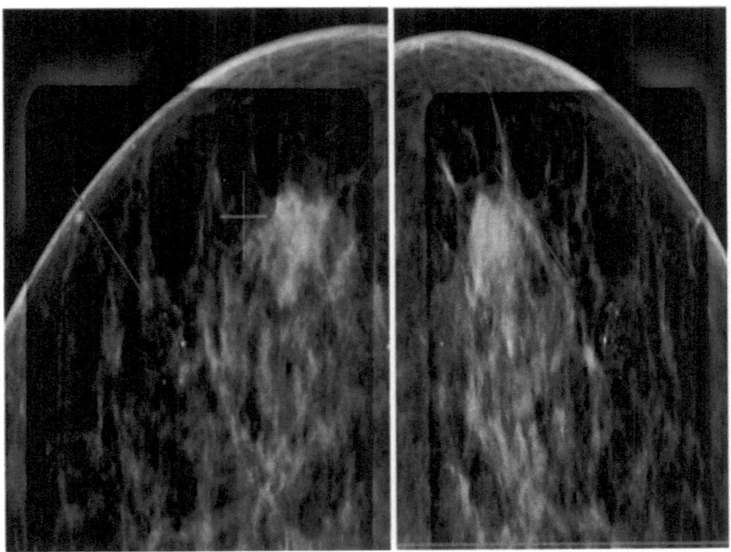

Figure 4b: Stereotactic views in stereo mode of a focus of microcalcifications at +15° and -15°.

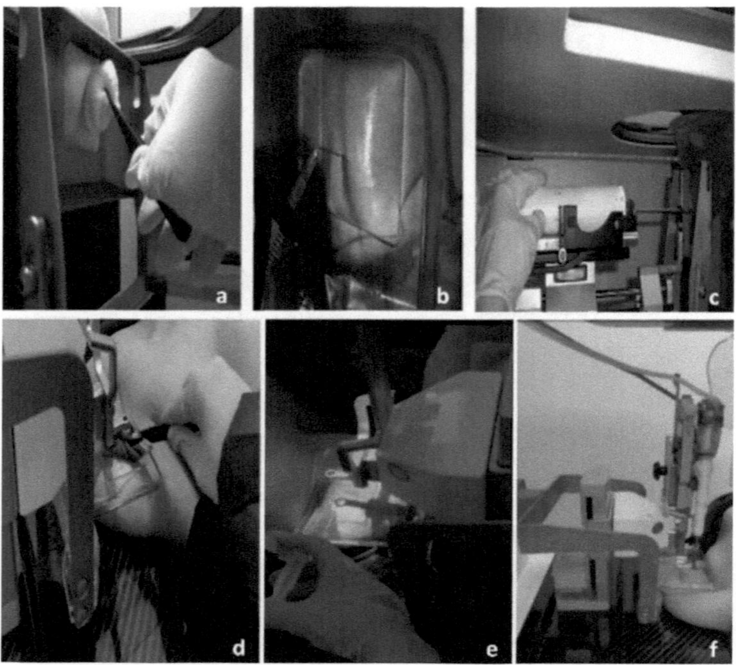

Figure 5. Stereotactic biopsy procedure on add-on stand

a. An antiseptic (betadine) is used to disinfect the skin of the breast, which is centred
and placed in the middle of the paddle.
b. Skin anaesthesia in the area of interest.
c. Placement of the needle on a dedicated digitised table.
d. Skin disinfection using an antiseptic (betadine) of the breast spread out and placed
in the centre of the pallet
e. Skin anaesthesia in the area of interest on an add-on stand.
f. Place the needle on the add-on stand.

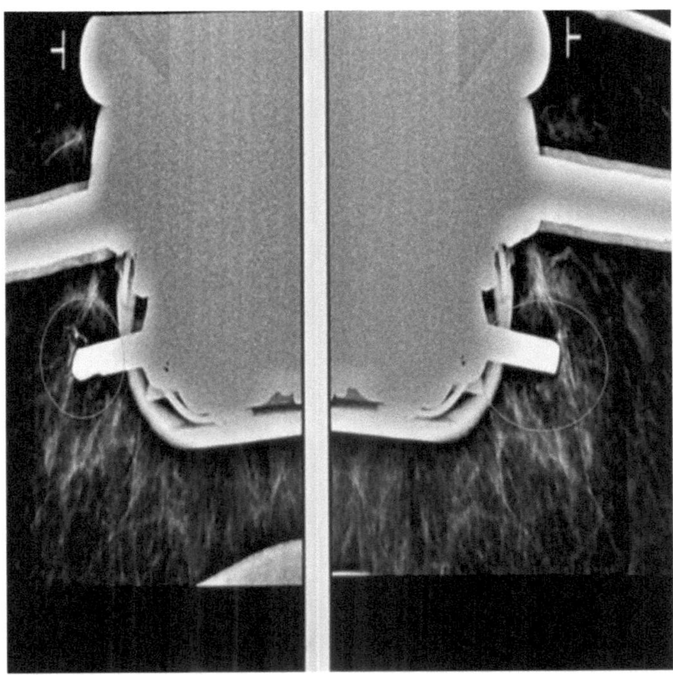

Figure 6. Pre-tir stereo images

➢ Pre-tir images taken in stereo mode (Figure 6);

➢ The needle is inserted using an automatic trigger system, and post-draw images are taken in stereo mode (figure 7).

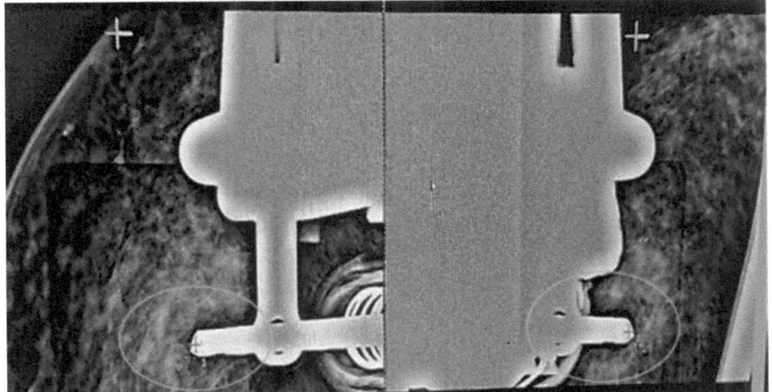

Figure 7: Post-shot stereo shots

When the lesions are microcalcifications, the samples are X-rayed to confirm their presence in the specimens (Figure 8).

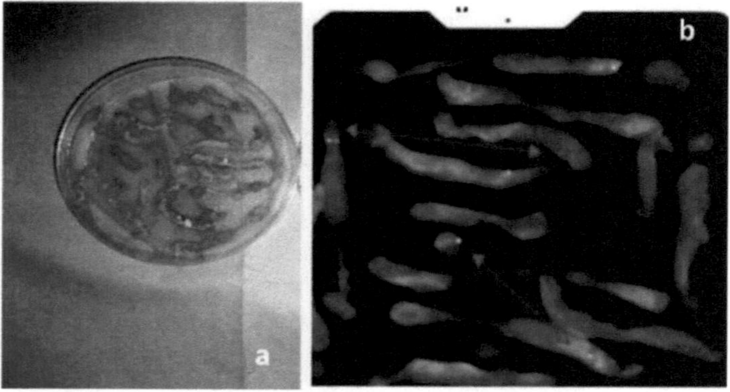

Figure 8: Specimens taken (a), X-ray of specimens (b),

4.3. End of the procedure

At the end of a stereotactic biopsy, if the entire lesion has been removed, a clip must be placed in the removal site to serve as a reference point in the event of further surgery, in order to optimise subsequent treatment (Figure 9) [15, 16].

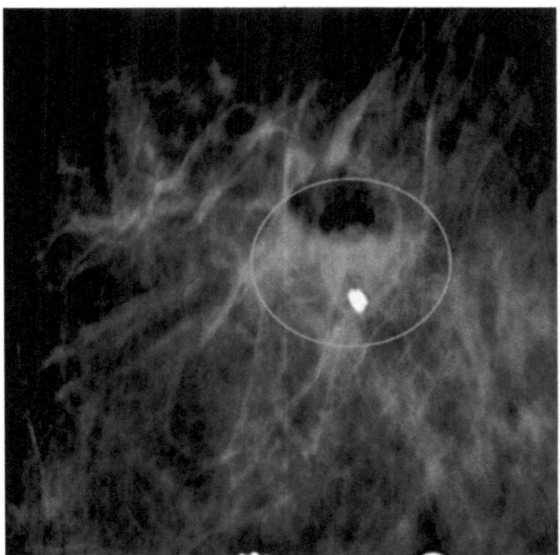

Figure 9. View of clip installation

It should be noted that the number of specimens will vary depending on the calibre of the needle, according to the ACR's international recommendations, with a minimum of twelve specimens when using large-calibre needles (7G) and six for smaller-calibre needles [9,12].

4.4. Post stereotactic biopsy

At the end of the procedure, the biopsied area must be compressed manually for 10 to 15 minutes, then a steristrip is placed over the incision and the wound is covered with a sterile compress, which is kept for 48 hours (an ice pack can be placed over the dressing without being in direct contact with the skin, to avoid and reduce the development of post-procedure haematomas). An oral analgesic may be prescribed for 24 hours (aspirin should be avoided).

5. Indications for macrobiopsy

Percutaneous sampling is recommended in three situations, see Appendix 1 (Figure 10):

➤ For highly suspicious lesions classified as BI-RADS 5, in order to optimise surgical management (therapeutic procedure);

➤ For suspicious lesions classified as BI-RADS 4, to avoid surgery on benign lesions (diagnostic procedure);

➤ For probably benign lesions classified as BI-RADS 3, in patients with homolateral or contralateral neoplasia or with the presence of risk factors (BRACA1 or BRACA 2 genetic mutation).

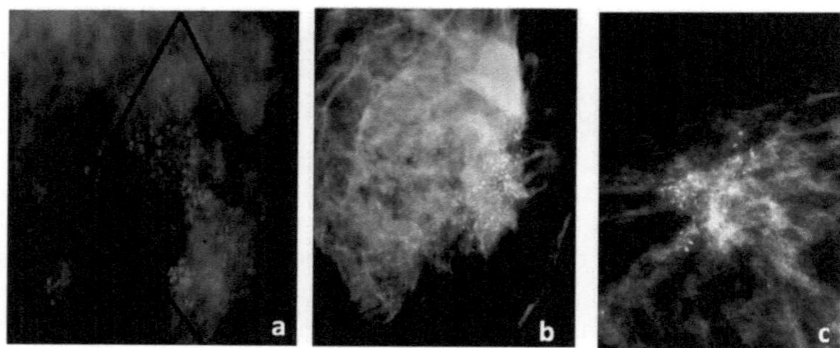

Figure 10
a. Segmental distribution of microcalcifications.
b, Linear distribution of microcalcifications.
c. Mass associated with microcalcifications.

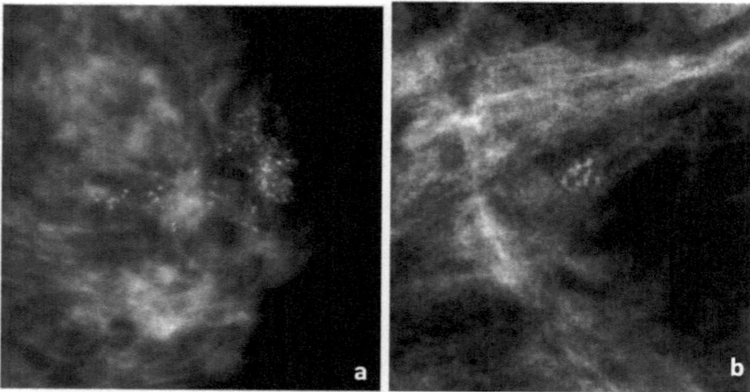

Figure 11. Microcalcifications classified as BI-RADS 4 (a) and BI-RADS 3 (b)

6. Contraindications of macrobiopsy

Abnormal haemostasis is the only contraindication to percutaneous sampling, as it is for macrobiopsy. If patients are taking anticoagulants, it is essential to stop them beforehand.

7. Complications of macrobiopsy

The complications encountered in macrobiopsy under stereotaxy are minor. They may include :

➤ Bleeding that can be controlled during the procedure and that subsides with manual compression;

➤ A small post-procedural haematoma (figure 12);

➤ Vagal discomfort, especially when procedures are carried out on addon systems;

➤ Neck pain for procedures carried out on a dedicated digitised table;

➤ Pneumothorax and distant infections are rare.

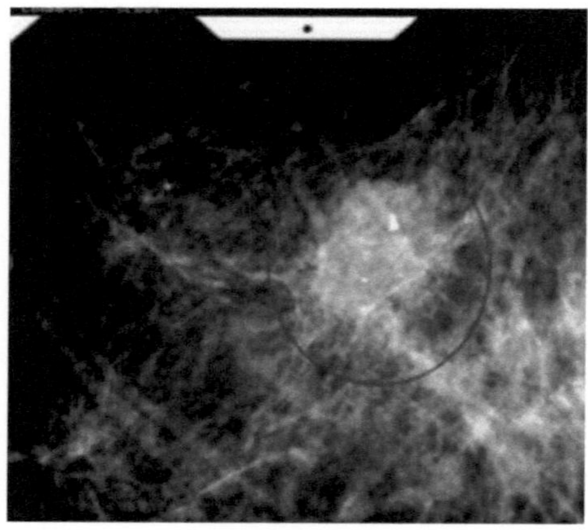

Figure 12. post-macrobiopsy haematoma.

8. Conclusion

Macrobiopsy under stereotaxis is an essential technique in the management of subclinical breast lesions, particularly microcalcifications, enabling a precise diagnosis to be made.

Message to remember

➢ Any subclinical mammographic breast image that does not show signs of benignity should be removed percutaneously;

➢ Macrobiopsy under stereotactic suction is a percutaneous sampling technique used mainly for suspicious microcalcifications.

Report of a macrobiopsy under stereotaxis

Date ....

Patient's name :
Name of prescribing doctor :
Indication:

Description of the target (microcalcifications, architectural distortion, mass visible only on mammography), its location and extent

Classify it according to the BI-RADS lexicon

Specify the gauge of the needle used

Specify the number of samples taken

X-ray the specimens in the case of microcalcifications and specify the number of samples containing microcalcifications in relation to the initial X-ray.

Mention whether the target has been partially or totally removed

Specify whether or not a clip is placed at the biopsy site

Specify the presence or absence of a haematoma

The report must be accompanied by an image including :

➢ A pre-procedure centring film (0°) ;

➢ Two pre-tir and post-tir stereotaxic images;

➢ A post-procedure centring photograph;

➢ An x-ray of the samples in the case of samples with microcalcifications.

APPENDIX 1: ACR BI-RADS CLASSIFICATION FOR MAMMOGRAPHY

➢ **ACR 0:** abnormality detected and awaiting diagnostic work-up;

➢ **ACR 1:** normal mammography ;

➢ **ACR 2:** considered benign (positive predictive value for cancer: 0%):

- Round masses with coarse calcifications (adenofibroma or cyst);
- Intramammary ganglion ;
- Round mass(es) corresponding to one or more cysts typical on ultrasound;
- Mass(es) of mixed density (lipoma, hamartoma, galactocele, oily cyst) ;
- Known scar(s) ;
- **Skin and vascular calcifications ;**
- **Large, clear-centred, parietal, milk-calcium calcifications, dystrophic, calcified sutures;**
- **Round, regular and diffuse calcifications.**

➢ **ACR 3:** considered probably benign (positive predictive value < 2%):
- **Round or amorphous calcifications, few in number, in small isolated round clusters;**
- **Small round or oval cluster(s) of polymorphous calcifications;**
- Few, suggesting the beginning of calcification of an adenofibroma;
- Well-circumscribed, round, oval or discretely polycyclic mass(es), without microlobulations, non-calcified, non-fluid on ultrasound;
- Focal asymmetry of density with concave boundaries and/or mixed with fat.

➢ **ACR 4:** are considered indeterminate (Positive predictive value > 2% and < 95%):
- **Numerous round calcifications and/or clusters of calcifications that are neither round nor oval in shape;**
- **Amorphous or dusty calcifications, grouped and numerous;**
- **Coarse, heterogeneous calcifications, few in number;**
- **Fine calcifications, polymorphic calcifications, few in number;**
- Architectural distortion outside a known and stable scar ;
- Non-fluid mass(es). Round or oval with a microlobulated contour or masked by normal or enlarged fibro-glandular tissue;
- Focal asymmetry(ies) of density with convex or evolving limits.

➢ **ACR 5:** are considered typically malignant (positive predictive value > 95%) :
- **Fine linear or fine branched calcifications ;**
- **Heterogeneous coarse calcifications or fine calcifications ;**
- **Numerous polymorphs grouped in clusters ;**
  - **Grouped calcifications, whatever their morphology, with a linear or segmental distribution (intra-galactophoric topography);**
- **Calcifications associated with architectural distortion or a mass ;**
  - **Grouped calcifications that have increased in number or calcifications whose morphology and distribution have become more suspect;**
- A mass with a blurred or irregular contour;
- A mass with a spiculated outline.

➢ **ACR 6:** lesions with proven malignancy (samples)

Classification of RTAs and Treatment and Advice (CAT)

CLASSIFICATION	CAT
BIRADS 0 (ACR0)	Incomplete work-up, needs further work-up
BIRADS 1 (ACR1)	Normal radiological findings
BIRADS 2 (ACR2)	Benign abnormality
BIRADS 3 (ACR3)	Probably benign abnormalities (follow-up)
BIRADS 4 (ACR4)	Suspected abnormality (biopsy)
BIRADS 5(ACR5)	Highly suspicious anomaly
BIRADS 6 (ACR6)	Biopsy-proven abnormality

CLINICAL CASES

Case 1

Patient aged 45 with personal history of breast cancer (left mastectomy).
Follow-up mammogram.
Normal clinical examination.

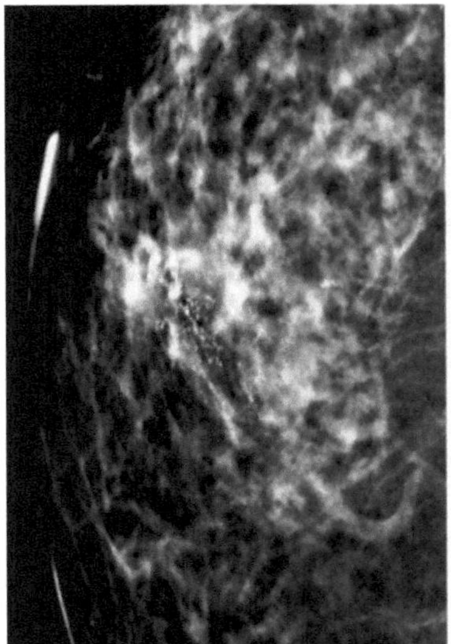 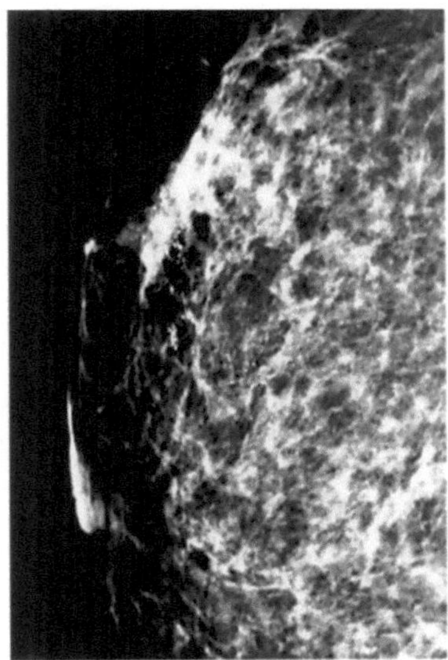

Figure 1: Right-sided incision.
Figure 2: Right oblique incidence.

Given that the previous mammogram was normal, what type of lesion do you detect and what BI-RADS classification do you propose?

Comments :

1. A complementary mammographic assessment: incidence profile and enlargement ;

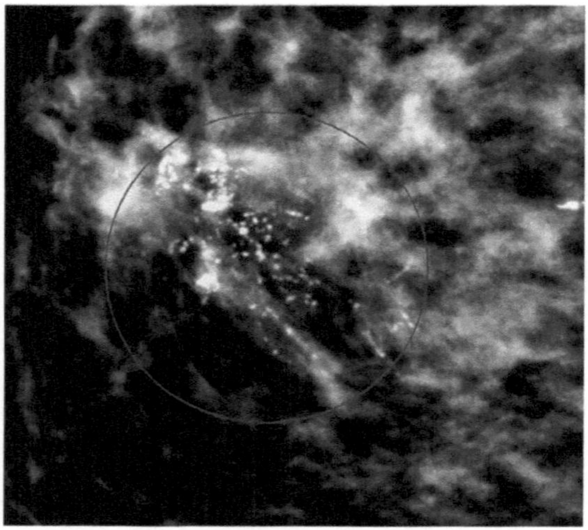

Figure 3: Enlarged view.

Confirmation of the suspicious nature of the microcalcifications, which were polymorphous, fine, amorphous and irregular, and of the ductal distribution, classifying them as ACR BI-RADS 4c.

1. A breast ultrasound was carried out, which came back normal;

2. Macrobiopsy under stereotaxis.

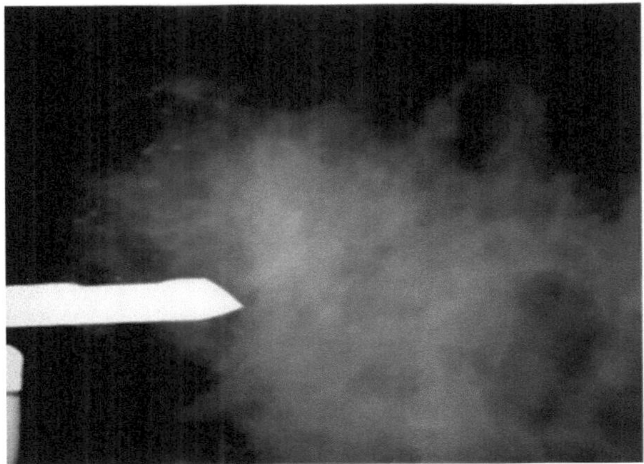

Figure 4: Post-shooting macrobiopsy image.

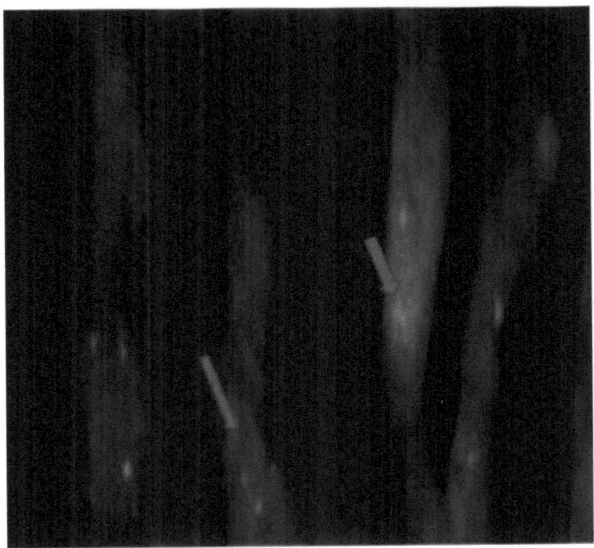

Figure 5: Radiograph of specimens containing microcalcifications (arrows).

1. Pathological findings: atypical ductal hyperplasia (ADH) ;
2. Perform a lumpectomy under stereotactic guidance (given the history and the risk of underestimation, which is 12 to 21% in the case of macrobiopsy for CAH);

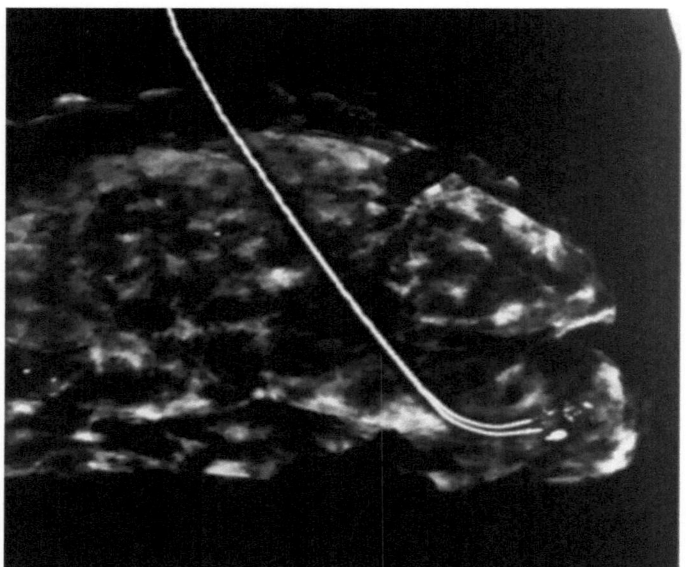

Figure 6: X-ray of the surgical specimen containing micro-calcifications after spearing.

3. Definitive pathology of the surgical specimen was consistent with low-grade ductal carcinoma in situ (DCIS).

Case 2

Patient aged 50, with no personal or family history of breast cancer, asymptomatic. Screening mammogram.
Normal clinical examination.

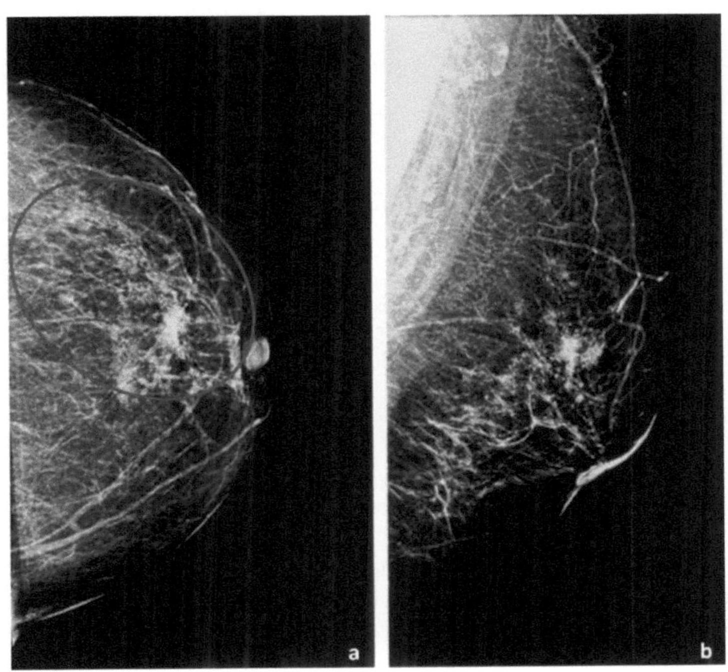

Figure 1
Front view (a) and left oblique view (b)

Extensive heterogeneous microcalcifications in the regional distribution QSE.

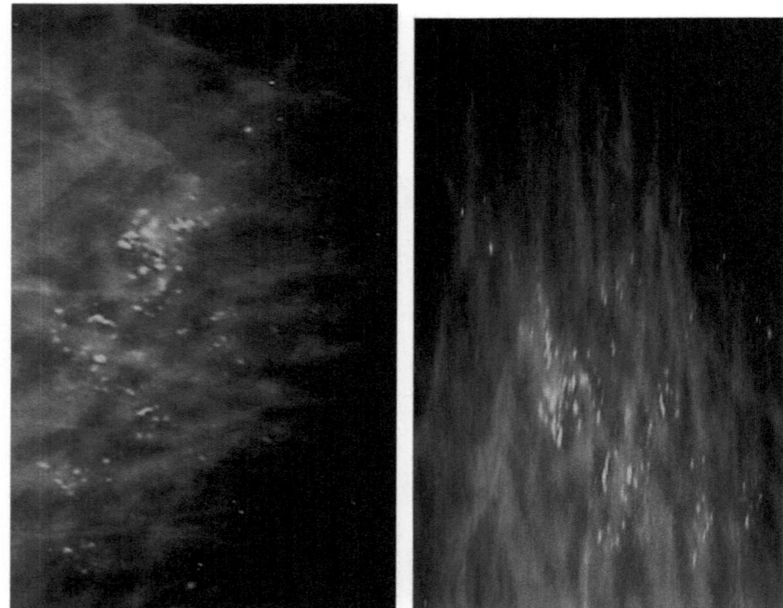

Figure 3: Frontal enlargement of the left breast.
Figure 4: Profile enlargement of the left breast.

Interpretation: mammographic analysis is in favour of polymorphic microcalcifications, not rounded, irregular, some linear, of regional distribution, classified BI-RADS 4b.

1. Macrobiopsy under stereotaxis.

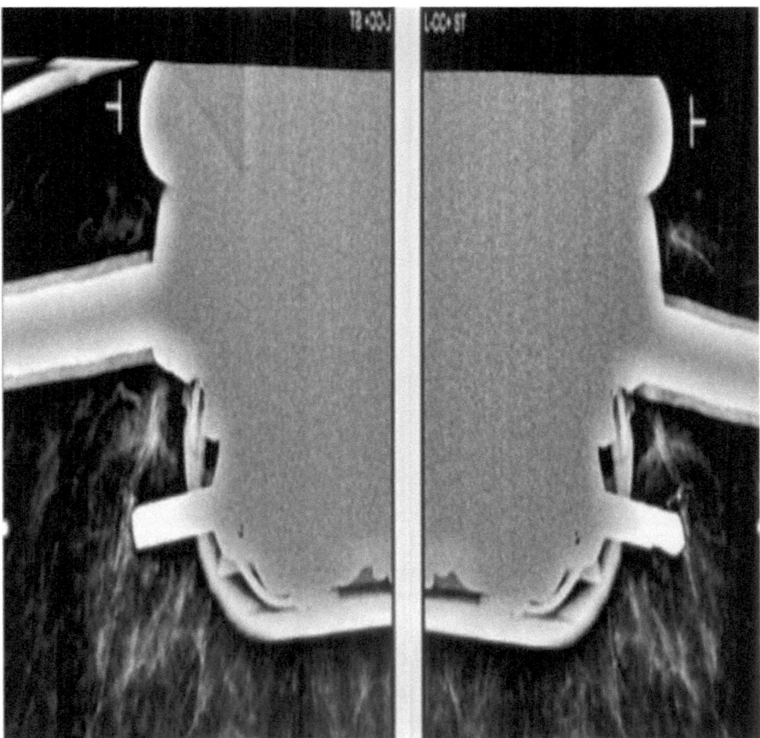

Figure 5: Cliche in stereo macro biopsy mode under stereotaxis.

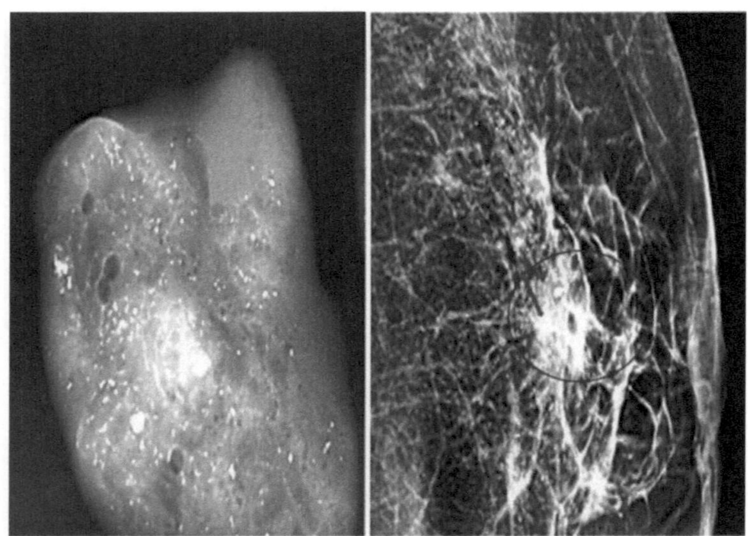

Figure 6: Radiograph of specimens.
Figure 7: Post-macrobiopsy image with clip in place.

2. Anatomopathological study of the specimens showed a non-specific infiltrating carcinoma.

REFERENCES

1. Willison KM. Fundamentals of stereotactic breast biopsy. Fajardo LL, Willison KM, Pizzutiello RJ, eds. Acomprehensive approach to stereotactic breast biopsy Oxford: Blackwell science, 1996; 13-72.
2. American College of Radiology, stereotactic breast biopsy accreditation program overview. available at www. acr. org.
3. Burnside ES, Sohlich RE, Sickles EA. Movement of a biopsysite marker clip after completion of stereotactic directional vacuum-assisted breast biopsy: case report. Radiology 2001; 221: 504-507.
4. Liberman L, Benton CL, Dershaw DD, Abramson AF, La Trenta LR, Morris EA. Learning curve for stereotactic breast biopsy: how many cases are enough? AJR Am J Roentgenol 2001; 176: 721-727.
5. Liberman L, Dershaw DD, Rosen PP, Abramson AF, Deutch BM, Hann LE. Stereotactic 14 Gauge breast biopsy: How many core biopsy specimen are needed? Radiology 1994; 192: 793-5.
6. Liberman L, LaTrenta LR, Van Zee KJ, Morris EA, Abramson AF, Dershaw DD. Stereotactic core biopsy of calcifications highly suggestive of malignancy. Radiology 1997; 203: 673-7.
7. Parker SH, Lovin JD, Jobe WE, Burke BJ, Hopper KD, Yakes WF. Non palpable breast lesions: stereotactic automated large-core biopsies. Radiology 1991; 180: 403-7.
8. Elvecrog E, Lechner M, Nelson M. Non palpable breast lesions: correlation of stereotactic large-core needle biopsy and surgical results. Radiology 1993; 188: 453-5.
9. Nath ME, Robinson TM, Tobon H, Chough DM, Sumkin JH. Automated large-core needle biopsy of surgically removed breast lesions: comparison of samples obtained with 14-, 16-, and 18-gauge needles. Radiology 1995; 197: 739-42.
10. Parker SH, Lovin JD, Jobe WE, Luethke JM, Hopper KD, Yakes WF, et al. Stereotactic breast biopsy with a biopsy gun. Radiology 1990; 176: 741-7.
11. Burbank F. Stereotactic breast biopsy: comparison of 14 and 11 Gauge Mammotome probe perfomance and complication rates. Am Surg 1997; 63: 98895.
12. Hagay C, Chérel P, Becette V, Gargay JR. Microbiopsies guided by digital mammography. J Le Sein 1998; 8: 38-45.
13. Hall FM, Storella JM, Silverstone DZ, Wyshak G. Non palpable breast lesions: recommendations for biopsy based on suspicion of carcinoma at mammography. Radiology 1998; 167: 353-8.
14. R Plantade. Interventional radiology: the cornerstone of senological

management. Journal of Diagnostic and Interventional Radiology (2013) 94, 591-609.
15. Ann surg oncol 2008 ; 12 j radiol 2008 ; 89: 40-6.
16. AJR 2008; 190: 949-54 Radiology 2001; 218: 407-502.

Table of Contents

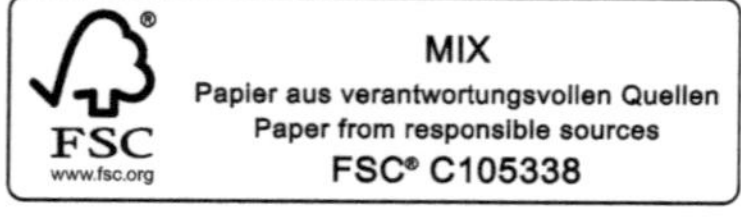

Printed by Books on Demand GmbH, Norderstedt / Germany